SHIPWREC
TO LYME BAY
FOR DIVERS AND SKIPPERS

Written by Nigel Clarke
ISBN 0 907683 59 2

With Grateful Thanks To
Nick Chipchase of Lyme Bay Deep Divers
Penny Hall

The book is dedicated to myself, as with out me it would not have been published. All the mistakes are by some-one else.

NIGEL J. CLARKE PUBLICATIONS
Unit 2, Russell House,
Lym Close, Lyme Regis,
Dorset. DT7 3DE
Tel: 01297 442513
Fax: 01297 442513

web site: www.njcpublications.demon.co.uk
email: mail@njcpublications.demon.co.uk

FOREWORD

This booklet has taken numerous hours of research and originally was intended to be used in conjunction with a chart. I have quoted the GPS numbers for all the wrecks listed and would be grateful for feedback on any errors. I also hope to update this booklet, and any further information about the wrecks such as the state of preservation would be most welcome.

Lyme Bay contains numerous shipwrecks, many of which have fallen into decay or been broken by the action of storm, salvage or demolition. Diving is one area where the amateur can be of great assistance to the marine archaeologists by recording and reporting any finds.

Many of the wrecks date from the First World War and contain unexploded ordnance items; these should not be disturbed - with the passage of time such items have become more unstable.

All wrecks host marine life; they have provided a refuge on a bleak sea bed, an oasis where life in a Spartan desert can flourish, but they also have the hidden danger of monofilament nets. Please beware of these nets when diving and always have knife.

Visibility in Lyme Bay is always a problem; the clearest wrecks are around Portland, but there you have the problems of tide. The wrecks near Lyme Regis and West Bay can be marine fog-bound in the spring - the algae growth which is known as "May Water". Storms also cause greatly reduced visibility; if you are travelling a long way, check out the weather forecast and conditions from a local dive shop, which should be able to advise you.

The layout of this booklet:-
Name of Vessel
Position (GPS)
Type of vessel
Tonnage - where known
Cargo - if known
Size - length x beam x draught
Date of sinking: Year/ Day/ Month.
Comments and additional information.

The listing of vessels is in alphabetical order; to see the rough geographical position please look at the map, which is not to scale and only gives the approximate location of the wreck, and from this the nearest port.

Some of the wrecks are more popular than others and many are fished by anglers. Knowledge of the tide times is necessary to dive nearly all the wrecks.

The Lost Wrecks of Lyme Bay

There are a number of vessels that were reported as missing in Lyme Bay and have yet to be positively identified or found. Information on these wrecks, or confirmation of identity would be most welcome and will be passed on to interested dive groups.

The Holy Grail of Lyme Bay Wrecks

Aeneas	10,049 gross tons	02-07-1940
HMS Amazon	1,081 Displacement	10-07-1866
Antigua Star	Motor Vessel	28-08-1922
Bayonne	2,589 gross tons	17-02-1917
HMS Bittern		04-04-1918
Borga	1,046 gross tons	01-03-1918
Chorley	3,828 gross tons	22-03-1917
Daphne	1,388 gross tons	11-11-1916
Enriqueta	145 gross tons	01-10-1911
Einar Jarl	1,849 gross tons	12-03-1917
Edison	469 gross tons	10-01-1894
Kingston Cairngorm	448 gross tons	18-10-1940
Kongshaug	1,156 gross tons	
Lesrix	730 gross tons	01-11-1960
La Blanca	6,813 gross tons	28-11-1917
Lord Stamp	448 gross tons	14-10-1940
M1 Submarine	1,600 displacement tons	12-11-1925
*N.Y.M.S. 383	260 disp tons	07-05-1945
Nerma	689 gross tons	25-08-1917
Naiad		16-08-1968
Osprey	426 gross tons	10-07-1866
Pergo	383 gross tons	01-02-1975
Polkerris	943 gross tons	04-03-1918
Quail III	162 gross tons	23-06-1915
Swanston	485 gross tons	20-12-1922
Sjaelland	1,405 gross tons	25-05-1917
Tandil	2,897 gross tons	12-03-1917
Veni	654 gross tons	10-05-1917
Willowbank	882 gross tons	22-12-1895

* N.Y.M.S. 383

This was a Norwegian mine sweeper which had the unhappy distinction of being the last vessel sunk in British waters by a German Submarine, after W.W.II in Europe had ended. The German Captain was unaware that a cease-fire had been signed. The U-boat (U1023) later surrendered at Portland Naval Base.

LYME BAY DEEP DIVERS

Lyme Bay Deep Divers are a group of specialist divers who, over the last ten years, have been investigating and recording wrecks in the 50-70m range in the area of Lyme Bay and out into the mid-channel. Interested divers are welcome to join this non-club group. They can be contacted via Nicholas Chipchase at 36 Scafell Close, Galmington, Taunton, Somerset. TA1 4LG Tel: Taunton 288872.

The group would also welcome and appreciate any information which would contribute to the ongoing research of the project. Information or details can also be sent to the publisher's address where it will be forwarded to the group.

PORTLAND DIVING

In recent years, and with departure of the Royal Navy, Portland has become one of the main centres for diving in the United Kingdom. There are several dive shops and numerous boats offering charter both in the area and across to France and the Channel Islands.

The area can offer a dive in all weathers, either within the confines of the vast Portland Harbour or the sheltered coves, and even has that rare commodity - some free public launching slipways.

Portland Harbour

The building of this vast harbour was begun in 1849, and continued through to the completion of the north eastern arm in 1905. It was built to provide a base for the Royal Naval Channel Fleet. The rock was quarried from Portland, and nearly 6 million tons of stone was used. Much of the labour was supplied by convicts. The harbour covers an area of 5,700 acres.

In the 1980's the Naval base was deemed to be surplus to requirements, and sold to Portland Ports. The last naval presence left in 1999 with the closure of the helicopter training base, though the Coastguard helicopter is still stationed there.

The commercial direction of the former harbour is not clear and some of the wrecks require a permit to dive on, although charter boats have their own permit. For further details please contact the Harbour Master for the Port. (Tel: 01305 824044).

Launch Sites

There are slipways at Ferrybridge, Castletown, Weymouth Sailing Centre and Weymouth Harbour.

Shore Dives in the Portland Area (see Portland map)

Newton's Cove:- Depth: 5-8 meters
Rocky ground best dived at high water.

Balaclava Bay - Grove Point Beaches:-
Depth: 12-30 meters.
Rocky ledges with lots of marine life. The tide near Grove Point can be strong.

Ferry Bridge Underwater Nature Trail:-
Depth: 5-8 meters
Variety of marine life can be seen. Dive slack water one hour after Portland H/W.

Chesil Cove:- Depth: 12-18 meters.
Large boulders and numerous bits of long lost wrecks can be found. There is little tide though the surf can make extraction from the sea difficult.

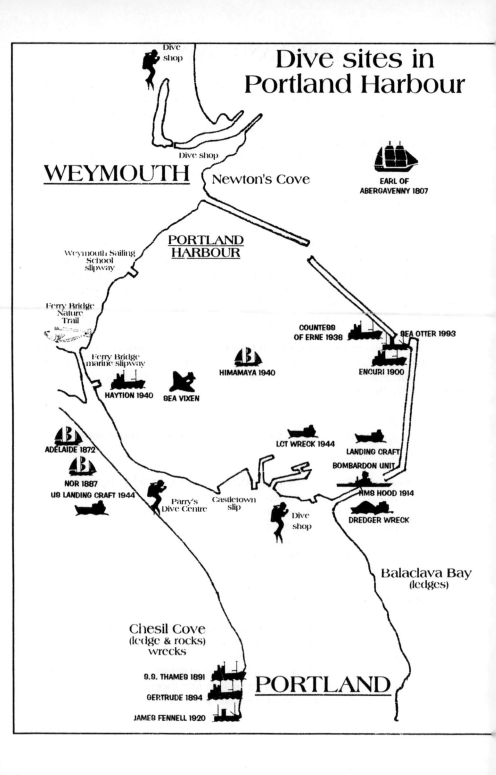

Dive sites in Portland Harbour

Dive shop

Dive shop

WEYMOUTH

Newton's Cove

EARL OF ABERGAVENNY 1807

PORTLAND HARBOUR

Weymouth Sailing School slipway

Ferry Bridge Nature Trail

COUNTESS OF ERNE 1935

SEA OTTER 1993

Ferry Bridge marine slipway

HIMAMAYA 1940

ENCURI 1900

HAYTION 1940

SEA VIXEN

ADELAIDE 1872

LCT WRECK 1944

LANDING CRAFT BOMBARDON UNIT

NOR 1887

US LANDING CRAFT 1944

Parry's Dive Centre

Castletown slip

HMS HOOD 1914

Dive shop

DREDGER WRECK

Balaclava Bay (ledges)

Chesil Cove (ledge & rocks) wrecks

S.S. THAMES 1891

GERTRUDE 1894

PORTLAND

JAMES FENNELL 1920

LIST OF SHIPWRECKS THAT CAN BE DIVED IN LYME BAY

AILSA CRAIG
Position: 50 33 68N 02 47 54W
Type: Steamship (armed)
Tonnage: 601 gross tons
Cargo: Coal
Size: 184ft x 28ft x 11ft
Date: 1918.15.04
Depth: 33 meters
The Ailsa Craig was an armed British steamer en route from Cardiff to Granville with a cargo of coal. The ship carried a stern gun and ammunition. The gun has been salvaged, though ammunition is still found. The wreck is now privately owned and is a popular dive. Around the wreck is an area of fine sediment, which is very easy to disturb if kicked up by a diver. The ship is reasonably intact.

ALGARVE
Position: 50 22 81N 02 48 51W
Type: Steamship (armed)
Tonnage: 1,274 tons
Size: 229ft x 34ft x 15ft
Date: 1917.20.10
Depth: 51 meters
The ship was torpedoed, killing 20 of the crew. The wreck was only positively identified in 1996, when the ship's bell was salvaged.

AMY
Position: 50 26 50N 02 31 26W
Type: Schooner
Tonnage: 230 tons
Date: 1928.15.03
Depth: 46 meters
The Amy was a two masted schooner that had been converted to look like a Q-Ship for making a film about Q-ships - the ship was sunk deliberately for the film. (Q-ships were ordinary-looking coastal traders that were equipped with the firepower to tackle a U-boat if attacked, during WW1).

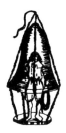

ATHEN
Position: 50 20 71N 02 27 72W
Type: Steamship
Tonnage: 2199 tons
Cargo: Patent crushed coal fuel blocks.
Size: 228ft x 38ft x 19ft
Date: 1906.19.02
Depth: 53 meters
The Athen sunk after an off-shore collision with the SS Thor of Cardiff. The wreck lies upright and the hull is intact.

AVALANCHE
Position: 50 26 56N 02 50 69W
Type: Iron Three Masted Sailing Vessel.
Tonnage: 1,210 tons
Cargo: General cargo (outbound Australia)
Size: 215ft x 36ft x 21ft
Date: 1877.11.09
Depth: 50 meters
The Avalanche was on passage from London to New Zealand when off Portland it collided with another ship, the "Forest", a 1244 ton sailing vessel. The damage caused sank the "Avalanche" within ten minutes. Of the 97 passengers and crew only 3 survived. The wreck was re-discovered in 1984 and a large number of objects were salvaged, many of which can be seen at Weymouth Museum at Brewer's Quay. The wreck is 20 miles WSW of Portland Bill.

BAMBURGH (see Gibel Haman)

BAMSE
Position: 50 26 25N 02 53 56W
Type: Steamship (Norwegian)
Tonnage: 985 tons
Cargo: Ballast
Size: 223ft x 30ft x 16ft
Date: 1918.17.04
Depth: 48 meters
The ship was on passage from Rouen for Swansea, and was attacked and torpedoed. It is broken up and lies 15 miles west by north of Portland Bill. The wreck has not been positively identified

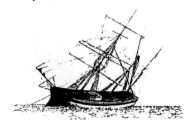

BAYGITANO
Position: 50 41 78N 02 56 07W
Type: Steamship (armed)
Tonnage: 3073 gross tons
Built: 1905
Date: 18.03.1918
Depth: 20 meters
The nearest large wreck to Lyme Regis and one of the most popular to dive. The ship was torpedoed during the First World War, with the loss of 2 crew. The U-boat captain then surfaced to ascertain which boat he had sunk. The Lyme Regis Lifeboat rescued the remaining crew. The wreck is broken up, though the bows and engines can be found very easily, and the boilers rise up and are very distinct. The wreck has been salvaged. The bows lie to the west. It hosts diverse marine life, and although it is fished all year, this does not seem to affect the large numbers of fish that can be seen. The mast lies off at an angle from the wreck, and is occasionally inhabited by a large conger eel.

BENNY'S WRECK (see MARGUERITA)

BERAR
Position: 50 41 90N 03 00 29W
Type: Barque (sailing vessel) Italian
Date: 07.10.1896
Blown ashore near Culverhole Point. The Berar was carrying a cargo of sawn timber and marble. The timber was salvaged by the construction of a raft and kedged back to Axmouth. The remains of the wreck can be seen at very low spring tides, though little now remains. There is a near-by wreck of a trawler called the Fairway. This was broken up on the beach though there are still some parts of it to be found.

BINNENDIJK
Position: 50 32 11N 02 20 01W
Type: Steamship (Belgium)
Tonnage: 6,873 tons
Cargo:
Size: 400 ft x 54 ft
Date: 1939
Depth: 27 meters
The wreck is very broken up and has been extensively salvaged. The vessel sunk after hitting a mine. The dive can only be undertaken during slack water. Visibility is often restricted on the site due to the nearby Admant Shoal and Shambles Bank.

BLACK HAWK
Position: 50 22 74N 03 25 31W
Type: Steamship (Liberty ship, USA)
Size: 441ft x 57ft x 35ft
Date: 1944.12.07
Depth: 50 meters
The ship was torpedoed and as a result of the attack the stern of the ship was broken off and sank. The forepart was salvaged and towed to Warbarrow Bay where it could be seen till 1967 when it was blown up to make way for a pipeline for the near-by nuclear power station at Winfrith. Shell cases and ordnance have been found on this wreck.

BLEAMOOR
Position: 50 22 .49N 03 26 15W
Type: Turret Deck Steamship
Tonnage: 3755 tons
Cargo: Coal
Date: 1917 27.11
Depth: 45 meters
The wreck lies east to west and is very broken up; at its highest point it is 7 meters clear of the sea bed.

BOKN
Position: 50 22 00N 02 59 01W
Type: Steamship (Norwegian built)
Tonnage: 698 tons
Size: 193ft x 28ft x 11ft
Date: 1942.09.07
Depth: 55 meters
The ship was torpedoed and sunk by German gunboats. The wreck lies upright but is very broken up. The stern section is reasonably intact but ends at the boiler. The wreck could be in two pieces. The winch and hold are aft of the engine. The identity has not been confirmed.

BOMBARDON UNIT (permit required)
Position: 50 34 33N 02 24 91W (see Portland map)
Depth: 15 meters
The Bombardon Unit was an experimental wave breaking barge which was star shaped. There are lots of hatches and girders. The wreck lies on a silty bed . Nearby is another barge with its rudder and propellers intact

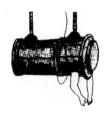

BOMA (Harold's Wreck)
Position: 50 32 18N 03 14 32W
Type: Steamship
Tonnage: 2,694 tons
Cargo: Potatoes, hay and straw
Size: 312ft x 39ft x 25ft
Date: 1918.11.06
Depth: 28 meters
The ship was torpedoed by UB-80. Extensive salvage took place during the 1970's.
The wreck is lying on fine sand and is very broken up. Visibility often poor.

BORGANO
Position: 50 26 15N 03 03 51W
Type: Iron Well Decked Steamship
Tonnage: 763 gross tons
Cargo: 1,000 tons of coal
Size: 195 x 30 x 14ft
Date: 30.06.17
Depth: 38 meters
The Borgano has not been positively identified. There is a confusion be-
tween the Lloyds loss chart position and that shown above. The vessel
rounded Start point at 5.30 a.m. in a strong NE wind. She was sunk three
hours later in a position WNW of Portland Bill.

BRETAGNE
Position: 50 29 50N 03 22 64W
Type: Schooner Rigged Steamship
Tonnage: 1439 tons
Cargo: Coal
Size: 232ft x 35ft
Date: 1918.10.08
Depth: 29 meters 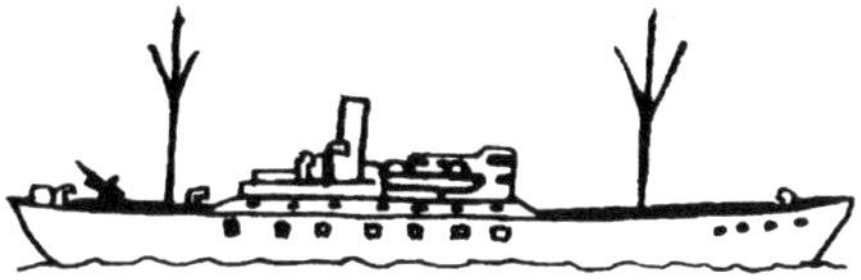
The ship was en route from Barry (S. Wales) to Rouen (France) when she
collided with another steamer in thick fog. She sank while under tow. There
was a stern gun in place, but this has been salvaged. There is still coal in
the holds.

BRITANNIA
Position: 50 20 31N 02 26 63W
Type: Steamship
Tonnage: 3028 gross tons
Cargo: General cargo and livestock
Depth: 56 meters
The Britannia sank after collision with another vessel. The vessel is very
broken up and the engine lies on the starboard side.

BRITISH INVENTOR
Position: 50 35 23N 02 18 59W
Type: Steamship (Oil Tanker)
Tonnage: 7000 tons
Date: 1940
Depth: 18 meters
The ship sank after hitting a mine. The aft section was salvaged and the wreck is now very broken up. The highest part of the wreck is only 2 meters.

BROOMHILL
Position: 50 27 61N 02 48 97W
Type: Collier
Tonnage: 1,392 tons
Cargo: Coal
Size: 243ft x 36ft x 15ft
Date: 1917.10.05
Depth: 47 meters
The " Broomhill" was scuttled after capture by a German U-boat. The initial gunfire killed 2 crew. The ship lies on her side and the propeller is missing. The vessel has been positively identified by Lyme Bay Deep Divers, who measured the hull to a length of 240ft. The wreck lies with the stern to the south.

BUESTEN
Position: 50 21 38N 03 24 47W
Type: Motor Sailor
Tonnage: 5187 Gross Tons
Cargo: Benzene and Kerosene
Size: 118.29 x 16.06 x 8.84 meters
Date: 09.04.1941
Depth: 50 meters
The Buesten was a Norwegian tanker that was sunk after bombing by the Luftwaffe. Twenty eight crew died in the attack. The wreck lies on the starboard side and the deck is vertical.

CHATEAU YQUEMS
Position: 50 29 11N 02 58 97W
Type: Collier
Tonnage: 1913 tons
Size: 280ft x 38ft x 21ft
Date: 1917.30.06
Depth: 45 meters
The vessel was mined or torpedoed while en route from Dunkirk to Barry in south Wales. The wreck is upright and the bows are NNW.

CHRISTMAS
Position: 50 39 38N 03 09 56W
Type: Trawler
Size: 57ft x 18ft
Date: 1981
Depth: 23 meters
The wreck stands 2m from the sea bed. The fishing boat sank while under tow in 1981. The wreck is off shore of a digger that lies abandoned on the beach. The digger was taken down to the beach to break up the wrecked trawler called the Fairway and drowned in the attempt!

CITY OF SWANSEA
Position: 50 28 86N 03 11 44W
Type: Steamship
Tonnage: 1,375 tons
Cargo: Coal 1682 tons
Size: 260ft x 35ft x 16ft
Date: 1917.25.09.
Depth: 39 meters
The ship was torpedoed and lies on her port side, with a detached stern section.

COUNTESS OF ERNE
Position: See Portland Harbour map
Type: Paddle Steamer
Tonnage: 900 tons
Cargo:
Size: 240ft x 30ft
Date: 1936
Depth: 14 meters
The steamer had been converted into a coal hulk and sank after breaking her mooring, on the inner side of the North Breakwater. Sea bed is silt and much of the super structure has been demolished. The wreck lies upright and can be dived at any stage of the tide.

DREDGER WRECK (permit required)
Position: 50 34 03N 02 25 45W (see Portland map)
Depth: 6-10 meters
This old sand dredger is very broken up. The bottom is sandy and tide here is not a problem . The vessel lies in two parts one section of 12m and the other 6m. The wreck is often buoyed and lies parallel to the sea wall.

DUDLEY ROSE
Position: 50 23 65N 03 26 42W
Type: Collier
Cargo: Coal
Date: 1941.09.04
Depth: 37 meters
The "Dudley Rose" was sunk after bombing by the Luftwaffe - the ship lies in an upright position. The visibility is normally poor on this wreck

EARL OF ABERGAVENNY
Position: 50 36 18N 02 24 39W
Type: Sailing Vessel
Tonnage: 1200 tons
Cargo: General Cargo and passengers
Date: 1805.05.02
Depth: 18 meters
The ship was captained by John Wordsworth, brother of the famous poet, and was en route for India. The vessel ran into the Shambles and became stuck. A small boat came out from Portland and took off 3 men and 2 women and a further 60 passengers were rescued as the weather deteriorated. Over 270 crew and passengers perished in the sinking. The wreck is about 1.5 miles SE of the harbour entrance. The wreck is covered in mud and there has been an archaeological dig on the site. You can still see some of the timbers and find musket flints.

ELANOR R
Position: 50 30 21N 02 20 72W
Type: Steamship
Tonnage: 4500 tons
Size: 370ft x 53ft
Date: 1939
Depth: 27 meters
The ship was mined and is located on the Shambles about 8 miles from Weymouth. The ship is very broken up and parts of the wreck are covered by the shifting sands of the Shambles. Beware of the strong tides in this area. The highest part of the wreck stands 8 meters from the sea bed.

ENCURI (The Spaniard)
Position: See Portland Harbour Map.
Type: Steamship (Spanish)
Tonnage: 3000 tons
Date: 1900.28.12
Depth: 12 meters
The Encuri dragged her anchor during a south west gale and was driven onto the breakwater. The wreck is now just a tangle of broken plates. The crew of 26 were saved from the disaster, but the captain and his dog went down with the ship.

14

FORESTER
Position: Inside Portland Harbour.
Type: Collier
Size: 97ft x 22ft x 9ft
Date: 1930.12.01
Depth: 10 meters
The wreck lies parallel to the harbour breakwater at Portland. The small
Cardiff based collier broke free in a storm and luckily drifted through the
Atlantic Royal Naval Fleet, before striking the breakwater and sinking.

FRANZISKA
Position: 50 28 36N 02 27 76W
Type: Iron Steam Ship
Tonnage: 669 net tons
Cargo: Coal
Date:1889.24.02
Depth: 55 meters
The Franziska sank after a collision with the barque "Honor Whist", while
on passage from Cardiff to Flushing. The wreck was identified with the
recovery of the bell. The ship lies upright and has a two cylinder engine.
The deck is mostly missing and the wreck stand upto 4m above the sea
bed.

FROGNOR
Position: 50 31 81N 02 33 44W
Type: Steamship (Norwegian)
Tonnage: 1,476 tons
Size: 260ft x 37ft x 17ft
Date: 1918.29.04
Depth: 35 meters
The wreck has not been positively identified. The " Frognor" was sunk by
German submarine (UB17). The wreck has been salvaged and is very bro-
ken up.

GALACIA
Position: 50 33 58N 03 26 37W
Type: Steamship (armed)
Tonnage: 5,922 tons
Cargo: General
Size: 400ft x 50ft
Date: 1917.12.05
Depth: 20 meters
The Galacia sank after hitting a sea mine. The wreck has been extensively
salvaged. The wreck lies on a sandy bed and there is a great deal of ma-
rine life.

GARM
Position: 50 16 58N 03 28 44W
Type: Norwegian Steamship.
Tonnage: 725 gross tons
Size: 54.63 x 8.53 x 3.81 m
Date: 1917.26.08
Depth: 55 meters
Torpedoed while en route from Liverpool to Rouen. Wreck lies upright NE-SW.

GEFION
Position: 50 30 10N 03 15 29W
Type: Steamship
Tonnage: 1123 Gross tons
Cargo: Coal
Size: 226ft x 37ft x 16ft
Date: 1917.25.10.
Depth: 32 meters
The Gefion was torpedoed while on passage from Penarth (S.Wales) to Rouen (N.France). The ship is broken up with the forward section lying on the starboard side.

GENERAL LEMAN?
Position: 50 21 30N 03 08 27W
Type: Trawler
Tonnage: 45 tons
Date: 1918.29.01
Depth: 52 meters
The trawler was sunk by gunfire and is very broken up. The highest point only 4m above sea bed. There is no confirmation with regards this wreck but the area consists of a great deal of debris. The site could consist of any number of trawlers sunk in this area.

GERTRUDE
Position: 50 32 80N 02 27 11W
Type: Steamship
Tonnage:
Cargo:
Size:
Date: 1994
Depth: 14 meters
The Gertrude was driven ashore during a storm. The wreck is very broken up and the boiler lies to the starboard side of the wreck. The anchor can be seen on the port side.

GIBEL HAMAN (ex Bamburg 1895)
Position: 50 35 90N 02 53 29W
Type: Steamship
Tonnage: 647 tons
Cargo: Coal
Size: 180ft x 29ft x 11ft
Date: 1918.14.09
Depth: 33 meters
The Gibel Haman was torpedoed by a German submarine and sank off Abbotsbury. The wreck lies upright but the mid section is very broken-up. The bows and the stern are intact and there is a gun pedestal on the stern.

GLOCLIFFE
Position: 50 27 11N 03 17 37W
Type: Steamship
Tonnage: 2,211 tons
Cargo: Coal
Size: 287ft x 44ft x 19ft
Date: 1917.19.08
Depth: 38 meters
The ship was torpedoed in an attack that killed two of the crew. The wreck is largely intact and lies on her port side. There is a gun, which is still mounted on the port side of the stern. The wreck is sometimes confused with that of the 16 ton trawler the "Irex" that lies close by. The wreck is on hard sand and rises 34ft from the sea bed.

GORIZIA (ex Glenmount)
Position: 50 25 80N 02 47 42W
Type: Great Lakes Steamship
Tonnage: 1957 gross tons
Cargo: Steel and brass
Size: 249 x 43 x 21ft
Date: 1917.30.04
Depth: 38 meters
The vessel was stopped by U-boat while on passage from New York to Le Havre. The Gorizia was boarded and sunk with scuttling charges. The wreck has been salvaged and is partially dispersed though lots of steel and brass remain. The brass cargo is in the form of 6" die discs which are 1/2" thick.

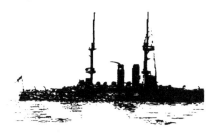

GRANE
Position: 50 29 38N 02 42 76W
Type: Steamship (Norwegian)
Tonnage: 1,122 tons
Cargo: Coal
Size: 231ft x 33ft x 14ft
Date: 1918 09.03.
Depth: 43 meters
The "Grane" was torpedoed by the German submarine (UB 80). The collier was on passage from Swansea to Rouen in France. The wreck is very broken up. The bell was recovered in 1986.

GREATHAM
Position: 50 18 25N 03 30 30W
Type: Steamship (freighter)
Tonnage: 2,338 tons
Size: 290 x 38ft
Date: 1918.22.01
Depth: 44 meters
The ship was torpedoed and lies upright and is very silted. The highest point on the vessel is 6m clear of the sea bed.

GRELEEN
Position: 50 27 66N 03 13 87W
Type: Steamship
Tonnage: 2,286 tons
Cargo: Iron ore
Size: 313ft x 38ft x 22ft
Date: 1917.22.09
Depth: 40 meters
Harland and Wolf built the Greleen in 1894. She was torpedoed, killing 19 of the crew. The bell has been recovered. The ship is now broken up.

GRETA C
Position: 50 21 53N 02 44 09W
Type: Freighter
Tonnage: 474 tons
Cargo: Granite chips.
Size: 170ft x 24ft x 9ft
Date: 1974.07.09
Depth: 51 meters
The "Greta C" sank in heavy seas when the hatches collapsed. One crew member was drowned. The wreck lies 15 miles south-west of Portland Bill. The vessel is intact and lies on the starboard side with the bows pointing south. The wreck was positively identified by Lyme Bay Deep Divers in 1996.

GRIPFAST (see Kingston Cairngorm)
Position: 50 25 98N 02 30 06W
Type: Steamship
Tonnage: 448 tons
Size: 161ft x 27ft x 14ft
Date: 1940.17.10
Depth: 46 meters
The ship sank after being hit by a bomb. This wreck was once thought to be the Kingston Cairngorm.

HAYTION (HAM)
Position: 50 34 68N 02 27 52W (see map Portland Harbour)
Type:
Tonnage:
Size:
Date: 1940
Depth: 8 meters
The wreck is very broken up and little remains except for the ribs and some old beams. The bottom is silt and there is a danger from sail boarders above

HAROLD'S WRECK (see Radaas)

HEROIN
Position: 50 40 52N 02 56 13W
Type: Barque (Sailing vessel)
Tonnage: 307 tons
Cargo: General/Migrants for Australia
Date: 1852.27.12
Depth: 18 meters
The ship sank during a gale. The crew and the passengers were saved by lifeboat and landed at Lyme Regis. The vessel was en route from London to Port Phillip (Australia). It was salvaged in 1853, and in 1994 bricks and other articles were salvaged by John Walker of Lyme Regis, using an air lift.

HIMALAYA
Position: 50 34 71N 02 26 59W (see Portland map).
Type: 3 Masted Steam Troop Ship (converted to coal hulk Coal Hulk). Built 1853.
Tonnage: 4,690 gross tons
Cargo: Coal
Date: 1941.12.06
Depth: 12 meters
The vessel had once been a troop ship and conveyed soldiers to the Crimean war. The ship was decommissioned and became a coal hulk in Portland Harbour. It was sunk during an air raid by the Luftwaffe in 1941. The wreck is inside Portland Harbour.

Diveable Wrecks in Lyme Bay

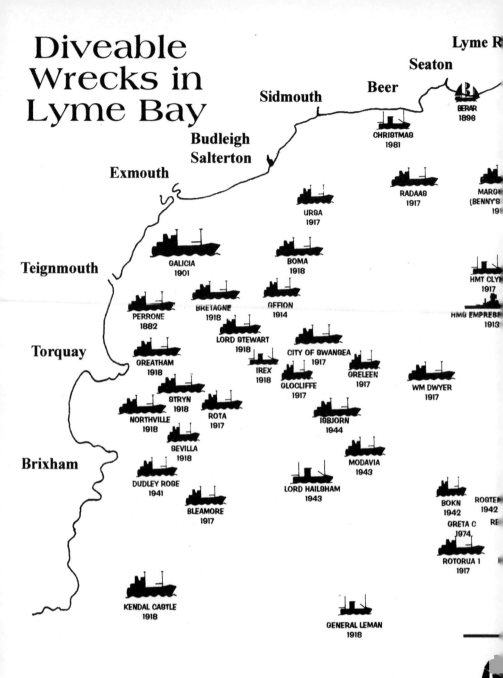

Lyme R

Seaton

Beer

Sidmouth

Budleigh
Salterton

Exmouth

Teignmouth

Torquay

Brixham

BERAR
1896

CHRISTMAS
1981

RADAAS
1917

MARG
(BENNY'S
19

URSA
1917

GALICIA
1901

BOMA
1918

HMT CLY
1917

PERRONE
1882

BRETAGNE
1918

GEFION
1914

HMS EMPRESS
1913

LORD STEWART
1918

CITY OF SWANSEA
1917

GREATHAM
1918

IREX
1918

GLOCLIFFE
1917

GRELEEN
1917

WM DWYER
1917

STRYN
1918

ROTA
1917

NORTHVILLE
1918

ISBJORN
1944

SEVILLA
1918

MODAVIA
1943

DUDLEY ROSE
1941

LORD HAILSHAM
1943

BOKN
1942

ROSTE
1942

BLEAMORE
1917

GRETA C
1974

RE

ROTORUA 1
1917

KENDAL CASTLE
1918

GENERAL LEMAN
1918

SAI
S

20

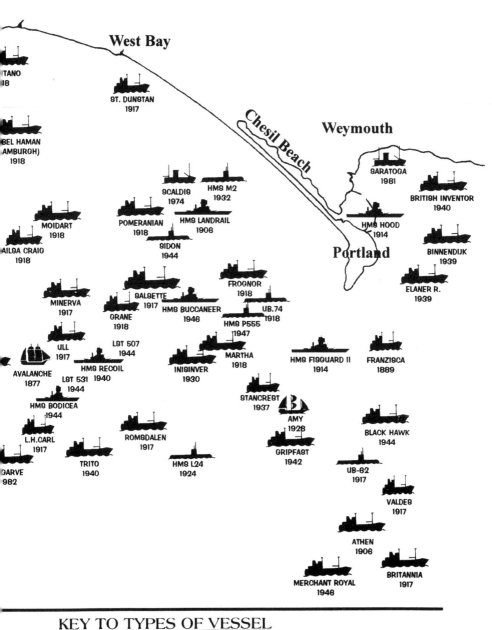

West Bay

Chesil Beach

Weymouth

Portland

KEY TO TYPES OF VESSEL

 SAILING VESSEL

 WAR SHIP

 TRAWLER

 SUBMARINE

SHIP

(All positions shown are approximate only)

HMS BOADICEA
Position: 50 25 66N 02 45 92W
Type: Destroyer
Tonnage: 1,360 displacement
Size: 323ft x 32ft x 12ft
Date: 1944.13.06
Depth: 50 meters

HMS Boadicea was attacked and sunk after an attack by the Luftwaffe during WWII. There was a large loss of life, with 75 crew perishing as a result of encounter. The stern section is upright and intact with four 7" guns. There are depth charges in the racks and torpedoes in the tube. The bow and bridge section are demolished. The bell has been recovered from the ship.

HMS BUCCANEER
Position: 50 29 36N 02 41 77W
Type: Admiralty Tug
Tonnage: 840 tons
Size: 163ft x 32ft x 11ft
Date: 1946.26.08
Depth: 43 meters

The tug was sunk while towing a target for gun practice. The wreck lies to portside and on the bow is three-inch naval gun.

HMS EMPRESS OF INDIA
Position: 50 29 75N 02 57 97W
Type: Battleship
Tonnage: 15,585 displacement
Size: 380ft x 75ft x 27ft
Date: 1913.04.11
Depth: 42 meters

The HMS Empress was used a gunnery target. The wreck lies upside down, and there has been some salvage.

HMS FISGARD 11
Position: 50 28 41N 02 29 82W
Type: Warship
Tonnage: 6,010 tons
Size: 280ft x 54ft x 23ft
Date: 1914.17.09
Depth: 68 meters

The vessel was the former Battleship "HMS Invincible". The ship sunk while under tow, with the loss of 21 crew. The wreck lies in a depression and is upside down. The hull stands 13m high above the sea bed. The stumps of the mast lie to the sides. Most of the teak framework has now been eaten away. The propellers and steering gear were removed when the ship was a training vessel. The wreck is a dangerous dive within an area of fast tidal currents.

HMS FORMIDABLE

Position: 50 13 23N 12 03 04 07W
Type: Battleship (built 1901)
Tonnage: 15,000 displacement tons
Size: 430 x 75 x 29ft
Date: 1915.01.01
Depth: 60 meters

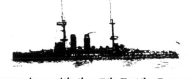

The Battleship was torpedoed while on exercise with the 5th Battle Squadron. Over 600 officers and ratings lost. The wreck lies upside down, with the hull mostly intact except for a split in the region of the forward funnel.

HMS HARSTAD

Position: 50 24 21N 03 01 41W
Type: Minesweeper
Tonnage: 258 tons
Size: 120 x 24 x 14ft
Date: 1943.27.02
Depth: 56 meters

The " Harstad" was a requisitioned former Norwegian whaler used as a mine sweeper during the Second World War. The whaler was attacked and sunk by German naval E-boats operating from Cherbourg harbour. The wreck lies with the stern upright and intact. The bows are on the starboard side to NW. On the bows is an attached Acoustic Hammer and gun bandstand on the sea bed. The wreck was positively identified by Lyme Bay Deep Divers.

HMS HOOD

Position: 50 34 14N 02 25 31W
Type: Battleship
Tonnage: 14,150 tons
Size: 380ft x 75ft
Date: 1914 04.11
Depth: 15 meters

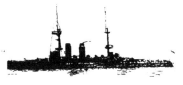

HMS Hood was sunk as a block ship at the entrance of the south channel to Portland Harbour, to prevent the infiltration of submarines into the Naval Harbour. The Hood lies upside down and the hull of the vessel is 2m from the surface at low water. The wreck can only be dived at high water or 4/5 hours before high water, due to strong tides.

HMS L.24

Position: 50 22 53N 02 37 91W
Type: Submarine
Tonnage: 1,080 tons
Size: 239ft x 24ft x 14ft
Date: 1924.10.01
Depth: 54 meters

The submarine sank after a collision with "HMS Resolution". The crew of 36 perished in the accident. The hatches of the submarine are open.

HMS LANDRAIL
Position: 50 33 75N 02 37 54W
Type: Curlew Class Gun Vessel
Tonnage: 950 displacement
Size: 195ft x 28ft
Date: 1906 04.10
Depth: 31 meters
"HMS Landrail" was a torpedo gunboat and was sunk while under tow after being used for target practice. The hull had been filled with cork which proved insufficient.

HMS LCT 381
Position: 50 23 46N 03 01 49W
Type: Landing Craft for Tanks
Tonnage: 350 tons disp.
Size: Capacity to carry five 40 ton tanks.
Date: 1943.27.02
Depth: 52 meters
Sunk while part of convoy (WP 300) after attack by German E-Boats. Wreck identified by Lyme Bay Deep Divers. The landing craft is upright and intact.

HMS M2.
Position: 50 34 60N 02 34 01W
Type: Submarine
Tonnage: 1,950 submerged Displacement
Size: 296ft x 25ft
Date: 1932.26.01
Depth: 35 meters
The M2 was lost with all hands, after a rapid sinking. The submarine was unusual in design and had hanger door to the front of the deck for launching a seaplane. The inquiry into the sinking blamed the faulty closing of the doors.

I spoke to an elderly mariner who had been on this vessel. He stated that: "the vessel had a tendency to kick back into the water when first breaking the surface. There would also be a competition to see how fast the crew could open the doors". Given the swell off the Chesil Beach it would seem a large volume of water rushed from the stern when the vessel surfaced and poured into the recently opened hanger doors. The vessel sank with all hands and is a designated war grave. The outer hull is now rotting and the props are missing. It is an interesting dive.

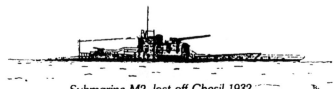
Submarine M2, lost off Chesil 1932.

HMS P.555
Ex US Navy S24
Position: 50 30 91N 02 33 52W
Type: Submarine
Tonnage: 1,062 submerged displacement
Size: 219ft x 21ft x 16ft
Date: 1947.25.08
Depth: 40 meters
The "P.555" was an American built submarine, which was transferred to the Royal
Navy under the "Lend Lease Agreement" of the Second World War. She was eventu-
ally decommissioned and sunk for use in the development of sonar, as a test site. The
wreck is in good condition.

HMT CLYDE
Position: 50 32 06N 02 56 36W
Type: Trawler
Date: 1917.14.10
Depth: 40 meters
The trawler lies upright and is well preserved though the wheel house and
some of the superstructure is missing. The vessel had been chartered as a
Patrol Mine Sweeper in 1915.

HMT LORD HAILSHAM
Position: 50 23 25N 03 02 84W
Type: Admiralty Anti-Submarine Trawler.
Tonnage: 445 tons
Size: 156 x 26ft
Date: 1943.27.02
Depth: 50 meters
Attacked and sunk by E-Boats while on convoy duty (WP300). The wreck
has been identified by Lyme Bay Deep Divers. She lies on the starboard
side with the bows to the south. Ordnance on the wreck includes numer-
ous rounds of 20mm shell and depth charges.

HMT RECOIL (ex German vessel Blankenburg)
Position: 50 26 41N 02 44 11W
Type: Anti Submarine Trawler
Tonnage: 344 tons
Date: 1940.28.09
Depth: 52 meters
The identity of the vessel has been positively identified by Lyme Bay Deep
Divers. The trawler was on anti-submarine operations, when it hit a sea
mine and sank. The wreck is upright in two sections, and contains depth
charges and shells.

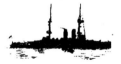

HMT REMINDO
Position: 50 26 16N   02 43 74W
Type: Admiralty Anti-Submarine Trawler
Tonnage: 256 gross tons
Size: 117 x 27ft
Date: 1918.02.02
Depth: 38 meters
The cause of sinking is not known and the wreck is thought to be that of the Remindo. The trawler lies upright and is broken in parts. There are live 303 rounds and a triple expansion engine.

INISINVER
Position: 50 29 40N 02 35 22W
Type: Motor Vessel
Tonnage: 126 tons
Date: 1930.09.09
Depth: 42 meters
The" Inisinver" sank after hitting a submerged object.

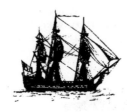

IREX ?
Position: 50 26 95N 03 14 64W
Type: Fishing Boat
Tonnage: 16 tons
Date: 1918.21.02.
Depth: 36 meters
The Irex was part of a small fishing flotilla which was sunk by German submarine. The wreck has not been identified and could be one of a number of other fishing boats sunk by gunfire in the same group such as "The Rosebud","The Leonora" and "The Onyx". All these vessels were sunk in the same area, and it is doubtful if any identity to the debris can be proved.

ISBJORN
Position: 50 22 70N 03 04 06W
Type: Steamship
Tonnage: 597 tons
Date: 1944.13.12
Depth: 56 meters
The identity of the wreck has been confirmed by Lyme Bay Deep Divers. The vessel lies upright and intact with little sign of damage.

JAMES FENNEL
Position: 50 32 76N 02 27 31W
Type: Trawler (Steam)
Tonnage: 215 gross tons
Size: 123ft x 22ft
Date: 1920
Depth: 15 meters
Steered onto the rocks during thick fog and an attempt at salvage failed. All the crew were saved. The wreck lies at 15m and is now very broken up and scattered over the sandy and rocky area.. The wreck is best dived when the wind is in an easterly direction. The wreck is 80m off shore opposite a window-like hole in the face of the cliffs to the north of Blacknor Point.

KENDAL CASTLE
Position: 50 21 56N 03 24 69W
Type: Steamship
Size: 352ft x 50ft
Tonnage: 3,885 tons
Date: 1918.15.09
Depth: 45 meters
The ship sank after being torpedoed. The wreck is upside down and her bows point north. The vessel sank with all hands.

KINGSTON CAIRNGORM (see Gripfast)

THE LANDING CRAFT (permit required)
Position: 50 34 37N 02 24 90W (see Portland map)
Depth: 12-15 meters
The landing craft wreck is intact and the bow doors are open but the vessel lies on silt which is easily disturbed.

LCT - The Tank Landing Craft
Position: See Portland map.
Depth: 17-20 meters.
The area is very silty, but the wreck of this W.W.II tank landing craft is intact. The vessel was part of the fleet for the D-Day landings.

L.H.CARL
Position: 50 23 98N 02 46 46W
Type: Steamship
Tonnage: 1,916 tons
Cargo: Coal
Size: 280ft x 40ft x 18ft
Date: 1917.20.07
Depth: 50 meters
The ship was torpedoed and now lies on its side broken up. The wreck rises to 6 meters in some parts.

LORD STEWART
Position: 50 29 61N 03 17 01W
Type: Steamship (armed)
Tonnage: 1,445 tons
Cargo: Coal
Size: 248ft x 36ft x 16ft
Date: 1918.16.09
Depth: 32 meters
The Lord Stewart was torpedoed by the German Naval submarine "U 104". There is a small gun in place on the stern. The wreck lies upright, but is broken in two. Phosphorus has been found on this wreck, which will ignite when dried on the surface.

LST 507
Position: 50 27 15N 02 43 59W
Type: Landing Craft (USA)
Tonnage: 1,652 tons
Cargo: Trucks and amphibious vehicles
Size: 326ft x 50ft x 10ft
Date: 1944.28.04
Depth: 47 meters
The landing craft was part of a convoy practising for the D-Day landings (Exercise Tiger). The convoy of vessels of which LST 507 was a part, was attacked by marauding E-Boats of the German Navy. The craft sank with the loss of 531 personnel. It lies NE/SW, with the stern N/ENE. The wreck is about 12 miles off Portland Bill. LST 507 lies in two sections, both upside down, and shows on the sounder as two separate wreck sites. The stern is SE.

LST 531
Position: 50 26 08N 02 44 79W
Type: Landing Craft (USA)
Tonnage: 1,652 tons
Cargo: Trucks, jeeps, armaments and soldiers
Size: 326ft x 50ft x 10ft
Date: 1944.28.04
Depth: 48 meters
Sunk after attack by E-boats, with the loss of 434 personnel, while taking part in operation Tiger. There is a small boat trapped under the upturned hull. LST 531 lies intact but is upside down with the stern section to NW. Research by Lyme Bay Deep Divers suggests that these identical vessels (LST 507 and LST 531) can be separately identified by the remains of the LST 531's forward boats which are still in situ. On LST 507 the forward boats were launched during the attack.

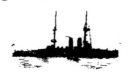

LUCINDA
Position: 50 25 93N 02 48 67W
Type: Wooden Schooner
Tonnage: 60 tons
Cargo: Mixed metals
Size: 79 x 16ft
Date: 1914.30.07
Depth: 52 meters
The schooner foundered 14 miles WSW of Portland Bill. Locally the Lucinda is known as the "Chain Wreck". The wreck was tentatively identified as the Lucinda by Lyme Bay Deep Divers in an uncharted position.

MAJORCA
Position: 50 20 20N 02 57 56W
Type: Motor Vessel (Panamanian)
Tonnage: 439 tons
Cargo: Bagged fertiliser
Size: 167ft x 28ft x 10ft
Date: 1982 18.09
Depth: 45 meters
The cargo of fertiliser shifted in rough seas while en route from Rotterdam to Teignmouth. The wreck lies upright, and is covered in nets. The ship's bell was recovered in 1993.

MARGUERITE (BENNY'S WRECK)
Position: 50 36 13N 02 58 72W
Type: Collier French
Tonnage: 1544 tons
Cargo: In ballast
Size: 260ft x 37ft
Date: 1917.28.06
Depth: 24 meters
The ship is also known locally as " Benny's Wreck", and is now a twisted pile of metal. Local boats regularly fish the area and there is lots of fish life. The highest point is 7.5m off the sea bed. The visibility is usually bad. The engine is on its side, one boiler on end and one horizontal.

MARIE DES ISLES
Position: 50 28 10N 03 16 72W
Type: Trawler
Size: 64ft x 20ft x 10ft
Date: 1980.14.11
Depth: 36 meters
Sank while under tow in heavy weather.

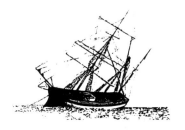

MARTHA

Position: 50 27 25N 02 38 17W
Type: Steamship
Tonnage: 653 tons
Size: 185ft x 27ft x 12ft
Date: 1918.07.03
Depth: 46 meters
The ship was torpedoed but lies fairly intact. Lies NE/SW.

MERCHANT ROYAL

Position: 50 20 08N 02 29 77W
Type: Freighter
Tonnage: 5,008 tons
Size: 401ft x 55ft x 26ft
Date: 1946.03.07
Depth: 60 meters
The ship's bell was recovered in 1984, though the name on the bell is "Goodwood". The ship sank after a collision. The vessel is upright and has been salvaged though much of this big wreck remains intact.

MINERVA

Position: 50 29 61N 02 45 41W
Type: Three Masted Iron Screw Steamship
Tonnage: 518 tons
Size: 182ft x 25ft x 14ft
Date: 1917.10.05
Depth: 45 meters
The Minerva was built in 1864 and was an early iron sailing steam vessel that still had the clipper sweeping bow with a flush deck. She was captured by German Submarine while en route from Caen and Swansea. The vessel was sunk with scuttle charges. There is a single compound engine. The identity of the vessel has been confirmed by Lyme Bay Deep Divers.

MODAVIA

Position: 50 24 41N 03 01 91W
Type: Cargo ship
Tonnage: 4,858 tons
Cargo: Aluminium, zinc, copper
Size: 400ft x 54ft x 28ft
Date: 1943.27.02
Depth: 53 meters
The ship sank after an attack by E-Boats, while part of a convoy. She lies on her side and has been extensively damaged in later salvage operations.

MOIDART
Position: 50 34 03N 02 47 29W
Type: Steamship (armed)
Tonnage: 1303 gross tons
Cargo: Coal and steel
Size: 243ft x 32ft x 16ft
Date: 1918.09.06
Depth: 33 meters
The ship was torpedoed amidships. The bow lies upright. The ship was on passage from south Wales to France. The "Moidart" was built in 1878. Parts of the mid-ships have been demolished. The wreck stands 8m high in places. The stern lies detached 15m to the south. There is a 40m scour under the bow of the wreck.

NOR
Position:
Type: Schooner with steam engine (Norwegian)
Tonnage: 943 tons
Size:
Date: 1887.18.01
Depth: 12m
The schooner ran aground in fog. The wreck lies about 100 meters south of the wreck of the Royal Adelaide. The wreck is broken up but if the pebbles are cleared away the propeller and shafts can be seen together with parts of the boiler.

NORTHVILLE
Position: 50 24 42N 03 24 48W
Type: Collier
Tonnage: 2,472 tons
Cargo: Coal
Date: 1918.17.02
Depth: 42 meters
Wreck lies upright and in good preservation.

NYASALAND
Position: 50 23 53N 02 53 74W
Type: Norwegian Steam Ship.
Tonnage: 383 gross tons
Cargo: Coal
Size: 148 x 26 x 9ft
Date: 1918.08.04
Depth: 55 meters
The ship was attacked by gunfire from U-boat 33 and sunk. The wreck has been positively identified by Lyme Bay Deep Divers. The stern is intact and lies to the north but the rest of the ship is broken up in the forward section

PERRONE
Position: 50 28 26N 03 22 87W
Type: Cable Layer (built 1882)
Tonnage: 3,342 tons
Size: 320ft x 42ft
Date: 1917.01.09
Depth: 26 meters
Sunk by a torpedo and is very broken up. The stern section lies alongside the starboard side.

POMELLA
Position: 50 17 86N 03 00 99W
Type: Motor Tanker
Tonnage: 6766 gross tons
Cargo: Crude Oil
Size: 457 x 57 x 31
Date: 1942.09.07
Depth: 59 meters
The vessel was part of convoy WP183 which suffered disastrous losses when attacked by German E-Boats operating from Cherbourg. The Pomella had an almost square shaped hull and the wreck lies on her side with the deck in the vertical position.. There is a deep scour below the hull. (see also Buesten).

POMERANIAN (ex Grecian Monarch)
Position: 50 33 58N 02 41 42W
Type: Liner
Size: 381ft x 44ft x 33ft
Date: 1918.15.04.
Depth: 35 meters
Torpedoed en route from London to Canada with the loss of 55 crew. The wreck has been salvaged. The ship lies E-W on its starboard side and in recent years there has been a great deterioration the structure of the wreck.

RADAAS (also known as Harold's Wreck)
Position: 50 34 25N 03 04 92W
Type: Steamship (Danish)
Tonnage: 2,524 tons
Cargo: Coal
Size: 290ft x 40ft x 20ft
Date: 1917.21.09.
Depth: 30 meters
The "Radaas" was torpedoed while on passage between Newcastle and Bordeaux. The wreck is very broken up and has become a haven for marine life. The identity of the wreck has not been proven but it could be the wreck of the Gallia.

REGGESTROOM
Position: 50 21 56N 02 57 56W
Type: Steamship (Dutch)
Tonnage: 2,836 tons
Date: 1942.09.07
Depth: 55 meters
The vessel was sunk after an attack by German E-Boats. The sea bed is a mixture of gravel and sand. The identity of the wreck is not confirmed and the wreck lies upside down.

ROMSDALEN
Position: 50 18 53N 02 44 79W
Type: Steamship
Tonnage: 2,548 tons
Cargo: 3500 tons of patent fuel blocks of crushed coal dust.
Size: 300ft x 40ft x 18ft
Date: 1917.17.02
Depth: 57 meters
The ship was torpedoed. The wreck is a large freighter and lies upright with thousands of coal dust fuel blocks still in the hold. The identity has been confirmed by Lyme Bay Deep Divers.

ROSTEN
Position: 50 21 71N 02 58 06W
Type: Steamship
Tonnage: 736 tons
Date: 1942.09.07
Depth: 56 meters
Wreck lies on port side and is twisted and collapsed. The wreck has not been positively identified. The vessel was part of convoy WP 183. Also lost in the attack were the Bokn, Reggestroom, HMT Manor, Pomella, Gripfast and Kongshaug.

ROTA
Position: 50 24 98N 03 18 92W
Type: Steamship
Tonnage: 2,171 tons
Size: 310ft x 45ft x 18ft
Date: 1917.22.07
Depth: 50 meters
The "Rota" was torpedoed and in recent years the ship's bell has been recovered. The wreck lists 20 degrees to the port side. There is extensive damage between the bow and the bridge.

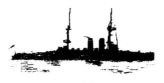

ROTORUA I
Position: 50 18 47N 02 59 73W
Type: Cargo Liner
Tonnage: 11,130 gross tons
Cargo: General
Size: 484 x 62 x 41
Date: 1917.22.03
Depth: 55 meters
The "Rotorua I" was torpedoed while on passage from New Zealand to London and is one of the biggest wrecks in the bay. She lies upright but has collapsed in many places. especially around the engine room. The top of the engine is the highest point of the wreck at 49m

ROYAL ADELAIDE
Position: 50 34 68N 02 28 59W
Type: Iron Sailing Vessel
Tonnage: 1,320 tons
Cargo: General
Size: 233ft x 38ft x 23ft
Date: 1872 25.11
Depth: 12 meters
This early iron sailing vessel was driven onto the Chesil Beach during a severe Southwest gale, on November 14 1872. The Royal Adelaide was on route from London to Sydney. All but five of the crew and passengers were rescued. The wreck lies about 100 yards off shore. (see Portland Map for position).

SALSETTE 1
Position: 50 29 68N 02 43 09W
Type: Liner
Tonnage: 5,842 tons
Cargo: General
Size: 440ft x 53ft x 30ft
Date: 1917.20.07
Depth: 43 meters
The liner "Salsette" held the 'Blue Ribbon' for the fastest crossing of the Atlantic and was owned by the P&O Shipping Company. The ship was torpedoed while on passage for Bombay from London. There is a gun mounted on the stern, and plenty of portholes still remain on the wreck. It is slowly deteriorating and the internal structure of the ship is starting to collapse. The masts have fallen alongside the wreck and the ship is in two parts.

SARATOGA
Position: 50 35 23N 02 18 59W
Type: Fishing Vessel
Size: 70ft
Date: 1981
Depth: 23 meters
The fishing vessel Saratoga sunk while under tow, only 4 miles from Weymouth harbour.

SCALDIS
Position: 50 34 28N 02 38 44W
Type: Trawler
Size: 80ft
Date: 1974.26.01
Depth: 35 meters
The trawler lies on her port side at an angle of 35 degrees. She sank during a storm with the loss of all hands. The hatches of the wreck are open.

SEA OTTER
Position: 50 35 05N 02 24 80W
Type: Trawler
Tonnage:
Size: 18ft
Date: 1993
Depth: 7m
The trawler sank in the small harbour that lies at the end of the breakwater near the Chequered Fort.

SEA VIXEN (JET)
Position: 50 34 74N 02 26 96W
Type: Naval Aircraft
Depth: 9m
This old naval jet was sunk for use in training exercises. The wings were taken off but the fuselage is intact. The bottom is very silt and easily disturbed.

SEVILLA
Position: 50 24 33N 003 22 96W
Type: Freighter (Spanish)
Tonnage: 1,318 tons
Cargo: Wine and fruit
Date: 1918.25.04
Depth: 44 meters
The vessel is known locally as the "Orange Man". The wreck lists to the port side at an angle of 20 degrees.

SIDON
Position: 50 32 93N 02 38 40W
Type: Submarine (S class) built 1944
Tonnage: 900 ton displacement
Size: 217 x 24 x 13ft
Date: 1955.16.05
Depth: 34 meters
The Sidon was badly damaged by an explosion caused by a malfunctioning torpedo, which exploded in the tube killing 13 of her crew on 16th May 1955, while moored in Portland Harbour. The submarine was eventually sunk as a sonar target. The Submarine lies upright and intact.

SIREN
Position: 50 12 40N 02 56 60W
Type: Iron Sailing Vessel
Tonnage: 1555 gross tons
Cargo: General, China clay in barrels
Size: 75.59 x 11.58 x 7.01m
Date: 1890.11.07
Depth: 60 meters
The wreck was identified by the recovery of the bell, in 1998. She sank after collision with HMS Landrail.

ST. DUNSTAN
Position: 50 38 28N 02 42 07W
Type: Enclosed Stern Bucket Dredger
Size: 188 x 38 x 15ft
Date: 1917.23.09
Depth: 27 meters
Commissioned as mine sweeper and sunk by mine. The ship lies upside down and is broken up, and rises 8m from the sea bed.

STANCREST (ex Shelldrake, ex Glenmor)
Position: 50 26 80N 02 32 50W
Type: Freighter (aft engines)
Tonnage: 462 tons
Cargo: Cement
Date: 1937.28.02
Depth: 46 meters
The cause of sinking is not known. The Stancrest sank while on passage from London to Bridgwater. The wreck was positively identified by Kingston BSAC and Lyme Bay Deep Divers. The bell has been recovered. The wreck lies on her side and is very broken up.

STRYN
Position. 50 25 04N 03 23 09W
Type: Steamship.
Tonnage: 2143 gross tons.
Cargo. In ballast
Size: 281 x 40 x 20ft
Depth: 40 meters
The ship lies on her side

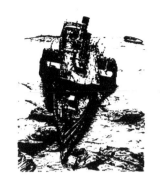

SUDON
Position: 50 30 98N 02 26 19W
Type: Steamship (Swedish)
Depth: 14 meters
The "Sudon" has been extensively salvaged and broken up and now lies
on a rocky sea bed.

THAMES
Position: 50 33 15N 02 27 15W
Type: Steamship
Tonnage:
Size:
Date: 1891 02.01
Depth: 10m
Struck the rocks and sank. There is not much left except plates and broken
wreckage. Visibility is normally good.

TRITO
Position: 50 23 03N 02 44 76W
Type: Steamship
Tonnage: 1057 gross tons
Cargo: Coal.
Size: 231 x 36 x 13ft
Date: 1940.20.09
Depth: 51 meters
The Trito was bombed en route from Port Talbot to Shoreham. Twenty-one crew killed.
The ship is fairly intact, but the bow is broken off.

UB 62
Position: 50 24 70N 02 26 00W
Type: Submarine (German)
Date: 1917.
Depth: 49m
The submarine was attacked by aircraft while on the surface, fifteen miles
out from Weymouth and sunk by torpedo. The U-boat lies at an angle of 45
degrees on the sea bed on her starboard side. The hull is holed.

UB74
Position: 50 32 03N 02 33 16W
Type: Submarine
Tonnage: 650 tons
Size: 182ft x 19ft
Date: 1918.26.05
Depth: 33 meters
The German submarine was depth charged and sunk by HMS Lorna.

ULL
Position: 50 28 00N 02 45 24W
Type: Steamship (Norwegian)
Tonnage: 543 tons
Cargo: Coal
Size: 168ft x 24ft x 14ft
Date: 1917.04.07
Depth: 50 meters
The "Ull" was torpedoed while on passage from Glasgow to Nantes in France. The wreck is very broken up. The vessel was identified by Lyme Bay Deep Divers based on the engine details.

URSA
Position: 50 28 18N 03 00 67W
Type: Steamship (Swedish)
Tonnage: 1,740 tons
Cargo: Coal
Size: 270ft x 37ft x 19ft
Date: 1917.17.09
Depth: 46 meters
The identity of the wreck has been confirmed by Lyme Bay Deep Divers. The "Ursa" was torpedoed while en route from Penarth (South Wales) to Rouen (France). The bows are smashed, and the galley of the vessel can be seen towards the stern on the starboard side. The wreck has been mistaken as that of the WH Dwyer.

US LANDING CRAFT
Position: see Portland map.
Depth: 12 meters
Date: 1944.13.10
Dive slack 2 hours after Portland high water. The vessel lies 90 meters from the shore. The landing craft sank in a gale after engine failure, and nine of the crew drowned. The wreck hosts a variety of marine life, though entry and extraction from the sea can be difficult if the sea is not calm.

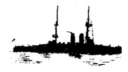

VALDES
Position: 50 23 70N 02 24 46W
Type: Steamship
Tonnage: 2,233 tons
Size: 265ft x 40ft x 17ft
Date: 1917.17.02
Depth: 50 meters
The steamer was torpedoed by German submarine. The wreck is broken up in large sections.

WH DWYER
Position: 50 21 06N 03 06 11W
Type: Great Lakes Steamship
Tonnage: 1770 tons
Size: 250ft x 43ft
Date: 1917.26.08
Depth: 55 meters
The ship was torpedoed on passage from Roeun to Newport (Wales). The ship was identified by Lyme Bay Deep Divers. The name of the vessel is on the stern, which is intact and lies to the north. The bridge, forecastle and deck have collapsed into the hull.

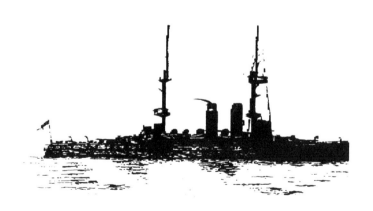